Praise for
Free and Clear

"*Free and Clear* is a wise guide to maximize your life and your space. When Karin's methods are applied, your mind, your home, and your life will feel lighter and brighter."

–Nadine Artemis, author of
Renegade Beauty and *Holistic Dental Care*

"Karin reveals how to break the declutter/reclutter cycle once and for all! She gets to the bottom of why we have this 'stuff' in the first place. An excellent read that left me motivated and inspired!"

–Amber Wientzen,
Founder, Lilac & Sage Classical Feng Shui

"This very practical approach to decluttering gets to the root of the problem—our emotional clutter in the form of unconscious beliefs. It brings a level of awareness to the issue that few books deal with and shows the way to finally get to the core of the problem in a step-by-step plan. I highly recommend this book to anyone who wants to take it to the next level."

–Alison Schockner,
Feng Shui Practitioner

FREE AND
CLEAR

7 Steps to Declutter
Your Home and Your Head

KARIN KISER

Camino
Chronicles
PRESS

Camino Chronicles Press
9450 Mira Mesa Blvd, Suite 320
San Diego, CA 92126

This book has been registered with the
Library of Congress.

Printed in the United States of America

To CK, with love,
who unintentionally inspired
my less is more approach.

Note to Readers

This publication contains the opinions and ideas of its author. It is intended to provide helpful and informative material on the subjects addressed. The strategies outlined in this book may not be suitable for every individual and are not guaranteed or warranted to produce any particular results.

This book is sold with the understanding that neither the author nor the publisher is engaged in rendering medical or other professional advice or services. The reader should consult a competent professional before adopting any of the suggestions in this book or drawing inferences from it.

No warranty is made with respect to the accuracy or completeness of the information or references contained herein, and both the author and the publisher specifically disclaim any responsibility for any liability, loss or risk, personal or otherwise, which is incurred as a consequence, directly or indirectly, by the use and application of any of the contents of this book.

Hold on!

Before you start reading, get your FREE gifts...

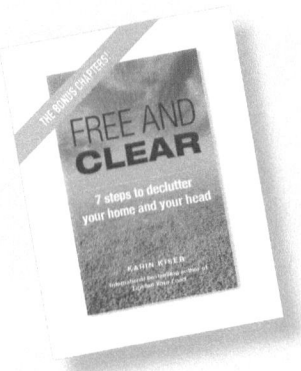

1. Clean Up Your Cleaners
2. Purge Your Personal Products

Each of these two bonus chapters will help you on your journey to be Free and Clear.

———✀———

To get them visit:
http://KarinKiser.com/free-and-clear/

CONTENTS

INTRODUCTION: DARE TO BE AWARE™

Clutter Is Not the Problem

If you've ever spring cleaned your house, cleared off your desk, cleaned out your closet, or donated some of your unwanted stuff to charity, you've experienced decluttering.

Declutter means to remove unnecessary items from your home or your environment.

Take a look around your house, right now. If you're like most people, you've accumulated quite a bit of new stuff since your last closet purging or trip to the donation center. What gives?

The problem is that your decluttering efforts were replaced by a gradual re-cluttering. Somehow, perhaps without your noticing, you accumulated just as much stuff as before, and your house is ripe for a bout of decluttering once again.

The truth is, your stuff isn't the problem. It's not even your fault. You've simply picked up the habit of re-cluttering.

This book will help you break the re-cluttering habit. When you break the habit of re-cluttering, you finally break free of the anxiety and exasperation that excess physical clutter can provoke. You become free and clear.

Now, if you are looking for the perfect method for folding your shirts or rearranging your stuff, this book is probably not for you. This book won't help you rearrange your current stuff in a new way. We often think decluttering means organizing. It doesn't. Yes, you can certainly rearrange your stuff so it is more orderly and visually appealing. But moving stuff around doesn't get to the real issue of why you accumulated all that stuff in the first place.

This book does.

Don't worry, you won't have to become a minimalist to massively benefit from this book. In fact, I'm not a big fan of the word "minimalist." I consider myself a maximizer. I live life to the max. I use my stuff to the max.

Using the 7-step *Free and Clear* system, you'll break the re-cluttering habit and experiment with being a maximizer as well. In doing so, you'll feel a renewed sense of freedom, appreciation, and ease with your external physical stuff and your internal state of being. You'll create some much-needed space in your home and your head, so you can have more of what you really want in life.

Have you ever heard of the 80/20 rule? Also known as the Pareto principle, the 80/20 rule states that roughly 80 percent of the effects come from 20 percent of the causes. That means 80 percent of your results come from 20 percent of your effort. In business, about 80 percent of sales come from 20 percent of a company's customers. You spend about 80 percent of your time in the same 20 percent of your home. This 80/20 rule applies to just about everything – including your stuff. We consistently use only about 20 percent of our stuff. You likely wear the same 20 percent of your clothes over and over. In *Free and Clear*, we take a look at the 80 percent you don't use so much.

In Part One: The Method, we dive into the 7-step *Free and Clear* system to decluttering. In Part Two: Putting It Into Practice, I'll walk you through how to use the system to declutter your closet, kitchen, living spaces – and even your mind. Yes, there is a mental component to clutter. If you've got physical clutter, chances are you have mental clutter too. They are related. Mental clutter is often at the root of your physical clutter. We'll get to the root cause of your accumulation – and set you free.

Here we go!

PART ONE:
THE METHOD

Step One

Awareness

The first step in the 7-step *Free and Clear* system is awareness. Why do you do what you do? Why do you accumulate excess stuff? What are the underlying thoughts and beliefs that got you here? This step is all about your WHY.

Before we dive into these questions, let's clarify what decluttering is and what it is not. The definition of declutter is to "remove unnecessary items." Decluttering is not just organizing or rearranging what you already have. Decluttering is simplifying.

The problem is that we often approach decluttering like we do dieting. We get inspired to tackle our closet or pantry, we donate a few bags of clothing to charity, and we feel pretty good about ourselves. That closet or pantry might stay clean and organized for a while, but eventually the clutter and excess stuff creeps its way back in. Before you know it, we are back where we started.

Same thing with dieting and losing weight. We get inspired by the latest juice cleanse or weight loss technique, we try it for a week or two, and we may even lose a few pounds. But then what happens? If you're like most people, your enthusiasm for cutting out all carbs or eating only grapefruit quickly dwindles, and – you guessed it – the weight eventually returns.

The missing piece in both of these examples is awareness – awareness of the deeper issue.

Let's be honest. There are lots of books out there offering tips and techniques to declutter your home. Likewise, there are countless ways to lose weight. But if you don't address the deeper issues – your underlying thoughts, beliefs, and behavior – the clutter returns.

Similarly with weight loss, if you don't fundamentally change your daily habits and beliefs around food (the things that caused you to put on the pounds in the first place), it is only a matter of time before the weight comes back. We've all experienced this.

Lasting change comes when you get to the root cause of the issue – the *why*. In Step One, we get to the why of your stuff. It is all about awareness.

So let's become aware of why we do what we do. Why do our efforts to declutter lead to eventual re-clutter? Re-cluttering happens when we are not consciously aware of why we buy and accumulate things. In my work with clients over the years, I've discovered that there are three root causes of clutter.

The 3 causes of clutter

1: The myth of more

As a society, we have bought into the belief that more is better. We want more time, more money, more business, more stuff, more "likes," bigger cars, bigger houses, bigger toys. The bigger the better! Supersize it! We are bombarded daily with more than 3000 marketing messages telling us that we need more stuff. If we want to boost our self-esteem, get the girl or guy, or be successful, more stuff is required. Even the government tells us that in order to be a productive member of society, we should buy more and consume more.

The truth is, more is *not* better. More is simply more − more things to take care of, more things to dust, more things to manage, protect, and insure. All of this more occupies both physical and mental space. It eventually wears you down.

It's hard to feel *Free and Clear* if you've adopted this cultural programming for more. It's not even your fault. It would be nearly impossible to grow up in this day and age without absorbing the belief that more is better. Everything about the current economic, societal, educational, and cultural system is set up to reinforce it.

Luckily, you can opt out. You get to choose what you believe. When you broaden your awareness, you may come to realize that more physical stuff isn't necessarily the recipe for fulfillment. Instead, you might discover the joy of other, non-stuff kinds of more − more experiences, more aliveness, more adventure, more connection. Not more physical stuff.

So when it comes to stuff, the critical question to ask is *why* do you want more? Why do you feel you need more? The answers to these questions are often related to the second cause of clutter.

2: Looking "outside"

At the root of why you want (or feel you need) more is often a direction imbalance. We often look outside ourselves for happiness and fulfillment, when happiness and fulfillment are essentially an inside job.

How many times have you said a version of this to yourself over the years?

- "If only I could lose 10 pounds, I would _____."
- "If only I were younger, I would _____."
- "If only I had more money, my life would be _____."
- "If only I reported to a different manager, I could _____."
- "If only I had more time, I could _____."
- "If only I had more help," _____.
- "If only I could _____, then things would be so much easier."

The *real* issue is very rarely the five pounds, your age, your boss, your family members, money, or time. The issue is that we look outside ourselves for an external solution to an internal problem. In other words, the reason we buy things is for the feeling that we envision those things will provide once we have them.

It's not about the external stuff. It's about the internal feeling that you think you will have by getting the stuff. In essence, you believe you will feel better by having the thing. If you've ever experienced buyer's remorse or the honeymoon effect, you know what I'm talking about.

Have you ever been excited about an impulse buy, only to wonder why you bought it a day or two later? What happened? Essentially you bought the *excitement* of buying it. It wasn't about the thing. Hence, the buyer's remorse.

Have you ever purchased an expensive piece of exercise equipment? You enthusiastically used it for two weeks – everything was great – and then the novelty wore off. Sooner or later it became a secondary clothes rack! That is the honeymoon effect at work. You bought the anticipated future feeling of being fit and energetic. You bought what you thought the object would give you.

We have all experienced scenarios like this, and yet, we go right on purchasing new stuff. Why? Because even though our past purchases have shown us that the stuff doesn't fundamentally make us happier or change our internal state over the long term, our mind convinces us that "this time it will be different." We fall for it every time. And so the behavior and resulting disappointment continue.

So how can you break this cycle? The first step is to realize that what you ultimately want is not the external thing per se, but the internal state of being or feeling you believe the thing will produce. That feeling or state of being could be a sense of security, success, value, love, abundance – you name it. So instead of looking outside of yourself for satisfaction or fulfillment, you break the cycle by changing direction and looking within.

You may be surprised to know that you can bypass the external thing altogether – and cut out the middleman – and go directly to the feeling. You can control your feelings.

Try these beliefs on for size:

- I have more than enough.
- I live in an abundant universe.
- I am enough, just the way I am.

You can choose to believe these things. I realize this idea may be uncomfortable for many of you. That's okay. Try it anyway.

Start asking yourself why you want the thing. Is it a need or a want? There's nothing wrong with wanting things, but *why* do you want them? What is the emotion or unmet need behind it? What's the underlying belief? Most of what we buy is based on emotion. Be aware of what emotion is driving you.

3: Distraction attraction

Do you allow stacks of mail to pile up? Do you let your desk become overrun with paper, magazines, bills, stacks, and projects? Then this third cause of clutter — distraction attraction — might apply to you.

Distraction attraction operates behind the scenes. You may not be consciously aware of this one. It's quite subtle. When your home or office is disorganized and cluttered, it is easy to become overwhelmed. This you know. What you may not realize is that there is a payoff to this disorder as well.

As a general rule, we only do things that work for us in some way. The payoff for clutter and disorder is distraction.

Distraction can promote a sense of busyness, of importance. Our minds and egos love it. Clutter also serves as a convenient way to distract ourselves from deeper issues — such as our feelings.

Obsessive texting or email checking, TV watching, internet surfing, video games — these may look like harmless ways to relax after a long day. They might seem like innocent ways to entertain ourselves.

The reality is, we often use these activities to numb out and avoid our feelings. We use constant busyness and surface distractions to avoid what's underneath, which in many cases is either a perceived void or an unpleasant feeling we would rather avoid. Sadness, dissatisfaction, frustration, anger, jealousy, worry all apply here.

In fact, we unconsciously create outer distractions to keep our focus away from our inner turmoil or perceived emptiness.

We do the same thing with food as well. Emotional eaters – and we all are emotional eaters to some degree – use food as a way to stuff our feelings and distract ourselves from what's really going on inside. The whole "comfort food" industry banks on this.

So the key here is to expand your awareness and consider what you might be trying to cover up or fill up with all this busyness and stuff.

Here's a clue to what might be underneath for you:

Imagine that your house were in perfect order. There's not a single thing extra or out of place. Your entire home is airy, spacious, pristine. Nothing to straighten, nothing to repair, nothing that needs cleaning.

Now imagine that you also have no to-do list. There are no emails for you to check, no errands to run, no chores to do, no appointments to keep. Really imagine that for a few seconds.

How would it feel? What comes up for you?

If everything were orderly and nothing (or no one) required your attention, what would you have to think about then?

Or how about this...

Have you ever seen those television shows about home makeovers or hoarders where a team of experts goes into someone's home and radically purges and changes everything? The home transforms from chaotic mess to model-home-like perfection in a manner of days. Are the homeowners ecstatic and overflowing with joy? Not always. Lots of them freak out. Big time. With no more external disorder to occupy their minds, they often begin to notice their internal clutter, which makes a lot of people uncomfortable – very uncomfortable. You might become uncomfortable as well. Notice how and why you might be generating unnecessary distractions and clutter for yourself.

When we become aware of why we do what we do, and become aware of our beliefs about our stuff, we have the ability to change them and break the re-clutter cycle.

Step Two

Direction

Now that we've broadened our awareness, we move to Step Two.

Step Two is all about direction. Consider the bigger picture. What are you moving toward in your life? What is most important to you? What do you value? If you had to rank these things in order of importance – family, friends, community, relationship, stuff, career – what would be number one? What about number two?

Where does your stuff rank?

Perhaps you're not sure what is most important to you. Maybe you don't have a clear roadmap for your life. That's okay. Let's clarify your direction with an exercise, shall we? Grab a pen and paper.

Let's suppose for a moment that you just received the news that you had only three months left on this planet. How would you spend your final 13 weeks? Who would you spend that time with? Where would you go? What would you do? How much time would you spend thinking about your physical stuff?

Visualize this for a moment and jot down whatever comes to mind.

Now imagine you got hit by a bus tomorrow and died instantly. Your close family and friends would be burdened with the unpleasant task of going through your entire house and all your stuff. All of it. Your papers, your sock drawer, your computer files, your garage, your storage unit, the trunk of your car, your secret stash of – everything.

What an eye-opener! For me, that thought alone was enough to inspire a new level of organizing, getting my papers and accounts in order, and simplifying my stuff.

Your time on this planet is limited. This is, by no means, a morbid thought. It is a fact. And it is a gift. You may be hit by a bus tomorrow, you may permanently check out in six months, or you may stick around for another 20 or 30 years. Who knows? The timing is a beautiful mystery! Embrace it! The inevitability of your physical death – and the mystery of its timing – are what make life exciting and meaningful right now.

So with Step Two of the *Free and Clear* process – Direction – we consider the direction we are going in our lives.

Where do you want to go with the limited time you have?

What's really important to you while you are here?

We are meaning makers

We know we can't take any of our physical stuff with us when we exit stage left. We all know this, yet we surround ourselves with stuff nonetheless. Sure, your children might want some of it, (again, the 80/20 rule) but your stuff really only has meaning to you. The stuff in and of itself has no meaning. We are the ones who attach meaning to everything. It's you who decides whether the physical objects in your home are important or not. Once you notice that you supply the meaning, you may realize that it's not about the stuff after all.

So why do we keep acquiring more? Simply put, we acquire things because we think we will feel better by having them. It's really not about the stuff, it's about the feelings you associate with the stuff. You think you'll feel better by having it. That feeling comes from within, not from the stuff.

For example, what inspired you to pick up this book? You want to declutter. Fair enough. But why? What is the feeling or state of being you want? You likely desire the feeling that decluttering can provide. Perhaps for you that means feeling free, peaceful, organized, empowered, calm, open, successful, clear. You want to go in the direction of what feels good. We all do.

You likely purchased most of your stuff for the same reason. You wanted to feel better.

The good news is, you can feel better now without having to link it to stuff. You can actually feel better, right now, by choosing a thought that feels better. Try it! It's the ultimate shortcut.

Break the link between feeling good and stuff

I invite you to pick a thought that feels better, right now.

I'm serious.

Whatever you were thinking just now, upgrade it to an even better thought. The topic doesn't matter.

Ready?

Go.

Notice how you feel.

If you do not feel better, try again. Experiment with an even better thought. It doesn't matter what it is about. It doesn't matter whether you believe it is true or not.

You have the ability to choose your thoughts and your feelings, 100 percent of the time. That's right. You are *that* powerful.

Unfortunately, most of us don't realize this. We are unfamiliar with our own power and the power to choose. We never learned this from our parents, from our teachers, or from our culture. Instead, what was modeled to us was the unconscious way of thinking and feeling.

Rather than actively choosing our thoughts, feelings, and overall state of being, we simply – and often unconsciously – react to whatever circumstances show up in our experience. This is backwards. A more empowered way is to consciously choose a thought that feels good, regardless of your circumstances.

Your circumstances don't dictate what you think or how you feel. You do.

So, what does this power to choose have to do with your cluttered closet or crowded living room?

Everything.

We buy things because we think we will feel better by having them. By actively choosing your thoughts and feelings on a consistent basis, you can break the link between feeling better and acquiring more stuff.

You can feel better with or without stuff. When you do this, you are no longer the victim of the declutter/re-clutter cycle. You are finally free and clear.

Fast track to the feeling

Let's practice choosing the direction of our thoughts and feelings.

Pick a thought that makes you feel better about yourself. It could be anything. Here are some examples:

- I am excited about _____.
- I am inspired by _____.
- I am grateful that _____.
- I am amazing.
- I choose to feel good.
- I deserve to be happy.
- I have a lot to be thankful for.

Identify one thought that can serve as your go-to, that you can turn to and remember whenever you need it.

Now, if you were to believe that thought and fully embody it, how would you feel? Feel that feeling now.

Practice this shortcut as often as possible. Start monitoring your thoughts. The moment you become aware that you start feeling badly, negative, or lacking in any way, stop immediately and change your direction. Remember the feel-good thought you just identified. Return to it.

When you can access this better-feeling thought on demand, you can easily release the stuff you once thought was responsible for the feeling.

When you change the direction of how you feel, the direction of your entire life changes as well. How amazing is that?

So to summarize, here's what we've covered in Step Two – Direction.

When you fully realize your days on the planet are numbered (and they are), you might not be as concerned about getting more stuff or holding on to all your current stuff.

Your stuff in and of itself has no meaning. You supply the meaning.

We purchase things because we believe we will feel better by doing so.

You can feel better right now by switching to a better-feeling thought or by visualizing something that feels good. You are powerful. Dare to be aware of your power to choose.

Before moving on

Before moving to Step Three, let's pause for a moment. What we've covered so far might have seemed a bit conceptual or "out there." I get that. As I warned in the beginning, this is no ordinary book on decluttering. Step One (Awareness) and Step Two (Direction) are actually the most important steps in the *Free and Clear* process. They are the foundation – and precisely what's missing in most other approaches to decluttering.

When you have greater clarity about where you are now and where you want to go, you can stop the vicious cycle of re-cluttering.

The success of the remaining steps is tied directly to how well you master Steps One and Two. These first two steps essentially declutter our heads. I recommend going back and revisiting them, especially when you are contemplating a new purchase.

Now let's move on to Steps 3-7 of the process, where we get to the nitty-gritty of simplifying your stuff.

Step Three

You Choose, You Use

In Step Three – You Choose, You Use – the goal is simple. Use your existing stuff. All of it. Remember the 80/20 rule? Now is the time to use that 80 percent. You might be thinking, "Now, wait a minute. Isn't the idea to get rid of some of my stuff?" Absolutely! But as I mentioned in the introduction, if you just get rid of a bunch of stuff without addressing why you acquired it in the first place, the clutter and excess will eventually accumulate again.

This is a critical step. This is what trips up most people. Most people periodically clean out their closets, clean out the garage, and donate piles of stuff to charity. Then six months later they have as much stuff as before – and oftentimes more – and the declutter/re-clutter cycle continues.

Luckily, you are not most people. You don't really need this constant stream of new stuff. In this step, we break the cycle.

Rather than throwing things away or rushing off to the donation center, we'll take the bolder approach of using our existing stuff first. That means you'll begin to use not just 20 percent of your stuff, but all of it. That includes eating all your food, wearing all your clothes, reading all your books. There are many reasons for this.

Reason # 1: When you decide to use what you already have, you become a smarter and more efficient consumer. You realize which purchases were useful and which were wasteful. You gain a deeper understanding of why you bought each item in the first place.

For example, what if you couldn't buy another cosmetic until you used every last bit of the ones you already have? You might think a wee bit longer about your next purchase before buying it. What if you couldn't throw it away either? Yes, that blue eyeshadow that's been sitting in the drawer for years that you thought would make a comeback. Now you must wear it.

Reason # 2: When you use your existing stuff to the max, you become a maximizer. You become more creative in finding uses for your stuff. Part of being a maximizer is realizing that there is no such thing as *away*.

Away does not exist. Americans generate more than four pounds of waste per person per day.[1] That's a ton of garbage every 15 months! That's also 60 percent more waste than our grandparents generated – and it's getting worse. Products that were once built to last are now intentionally designed with built-in obsolescence – meaning, when they break (not *if* they break, but *when* they break), it will be much cheaper to get a new one than to repair it. So now the norm is to "throw it out and get a new one."

The daily marketing messages we receive reinforce this new "just get a new one" habit. Our society – including our peers, co-workers, friends, and family – also contribute to this behavior. Somehow if your phone is more than three years old, you're considered a dinosaur who is behind the times and out of touch. We've become a throw-away society. Unfortunately, away doesn't exist. When you throw something away, it doesn't just vanish into nothingness. It only relocates. It was once in your closet, garage, or office, and now it is relocated to a landfill, incinerator, or ocean. Not good. So in this step, you use your existing stuff. Starting now.

Step Four

Press Pause

Step Four of the *Free and Clear* process is simple. Stop buying stuff. This step goes hand in hand with the previous one. Once you accept the challenge to use your existing stuff, there's no need to rush out and buy anything new. So, temporarily press the pause button on all new purchases.

See how long you can go without buying anything. Make a game out of it. Start with food. How long can you go just eating the food you already have? Have fun with it! Actually use all your sauces and spices. You might be surprised by how many creative new dishes and combinations you can come up with.

Now see how long you can go before buying a new item of clothing. You already have plenty of clothes. Right now you're only wearing about 20 percent of your wardrobe anyway, so in essence, you can go shopping in the other 80 percent of your closet!

You might be wondering, "What's the point of these exercises?" The main point is to break the consumption habit. Another reason is to see what's underneath it — what's at the root of the habit. For example, if I were to suggest that you refrain from buying *anything* for two months, what comes up for you? Notice whatever thought pops into your head. Notice how you are feeling.

Many of us have mistakenly linked our sense of self-worth and value to our physical stuff. This exercise is the fast-track way to realize if this is true for you. If you feel anxious, negative, or uncomfortable in any way about the idea of not buying stuff, it's quite possible you have a limiting belief or two that's been stored in your subconscious mind.

Examples of limiting beliefs around stuff include:

- It's better to be safe than sorry.

- Bigger is better.

- Any sentence that starts with "I should…"

- Any sentence that begins with "I can't…"

- Sentences that include a "if only I could…"

Replace any limiting, outdated, or disempowering beliefs with one or more of these:

- I am enough.

- I have more than enough.

- I am grateful for all that I have.

- I am grateful for all the abundance that surrounds me now.

- I am a maximizer.

- I deserve to be free and clear.

- I am at peace with myself now.

- Fulfillment comes from within me.

- I accept and appreciate myself.

- I can choose a better-feeling thought.

- I take full responsibility for my life.

Being grateful, feeling worthy, and adopting new, supportive beliefs are all powerful ways to break the consumption habit. When you temporarily press pause on new purchases and maximize your current stuff, you also unplug from the mainstream that says you need to be constantly buying and accumulating more to be a worthy member of society. You are worthy already!

Onward to Step Five.

Step Five

Lay It Out

It's a lot easier to use all of your current stuff – the 80 and the 20 – if you can see it. That means pulling out things that are hiding in cabinets, closets, and drawers and laying them out in plain view.

Yes, I realize doing this will make your home seem even more cluttered. That's okay. It's temporary. However, to avoid feeling overwhelmed, let's start with something small, like a drawer or medicine cabinet in your bathroom.

Take everything out of that drawer or medicine cabinet and spread it out on the bathroom counter. The drawer or cabinet should now be completely empty. Use this opportunity to thoroughly clean or dust the inside of it.

Now, start using your stuff.

Only put something back in the cabinet or drawer *after* you have actually used it.

The goal of this exercise is to step back and actually SEE all your stuff. It can be eye-opening for two reasons. On the one hand, just look at all the abundance in front of you! Take it all in and feel grateful for all the physical abundance you currently enjoy. On the other hand, your eyes might be opening now to just how many things you have but rarely use.

If three weeks go by and you still haven't used that blue eyeshadow from the 90s or the cologne you received as a gift, consider passing them on to people who *will* use them.

Step Six

The Six Questions

In Step Six, we use six questions to determine what to keep and what to recycle. The goal is to identify the 20 percent of your stuff that adds joy, utility, or convenience to your life – and to simplify the rest.

Here are the questions:

Question # 1: "Are there any negative feelings or memories associated with this item?"

Question # 2: "Do I regularly use this item?"

Question # 3: "Have I used it in the last six months?"

Question # 4: "Does this item positively contribute to my life?"

Question # 5: "Am I keeping this because I think I *might* use it at some point?"

Question # 6: "Am I keeping it out of guilt?"

Let's go back to the medicine cabinet example and see how we might apply the six questions.

1: Negativity

"Are there any negative feelings or memories associated with anything in this medicine cabinet?"

Possible response: "Well, there's the expired prescription I took when my back went out. I thought I would hold onto it just in case."

Red alert!

The idea of throwing your back out – and entertaining the possibility of a recurrence – definitely qualifies as a negative association. Best to return the prescription to the pharmacy for proper disposal.

2: Regularity

"Do I regularly use this item?"

Possible response: Just a "yes" or "no" will do.

3: Utility

"Have I used it in the last six months?"

Possible response: "Nope, I have not used this lipstick in years."

Now's your chance! Keep that lipstick on the counter for the next three weeks as a daily reminder to use it. If three weeks go by and you still haven't used it, it's time to pass it along to someone who will (after properly sterilizing it, of course).

4: Contribution

"Does this item positively contribute to my life?" In other words, do you feel good when you use it?

Possible response: "I liked this lotion/deodorant/cologne when I bought it, but after using it a few times, I realized it was too strong for me."

5: Might

"Am I keeping this because I think I might use it at some point?"

For anything that is a "might," keep it on the counter where you can see it. You'll know soon enough if you will use it or you won't.

6: Guilt

"Am I keeping it out of guilt?"

Guilt tends to creep in when the item in question was a gift, when we associate it with waste (for example, when we spent a lot of money on it), and when it was an impulse buy.

Step Seven

Repurpose or Recycle

Once you've identified items that you're not using and that no longer positively contribute to your life, it's time to repurpose or recycle them. In our medicine cabinet example, who else might benefit from that lotion or cologne you're not using? Perhaps your friends or family members might want them. Check to see if any women's shelters in your area accept unopened or gently used items.

If you can't find a new home for the personal products you aren't using, what part of them can be recycled? Can the paper, plastic, or glass in the packaging be recycled? Remember, there is no such thing as *away* when you throw something out. Only dispose of it in the trash as a last resort.

PART TWO: PUTTING IT INTO PRACTICE

In Part Two, we'll apply the 7-step *Free and Clear* method to different areas of your home. But before you head straight to your bedroom closet, let's start with something a bit smaller. That way you can get a feel for the process and experience an immediate win.

Let's start with your wallet, purse, or whatever you have in your pockets right now. Here goes...

Step One: Awareness

This step is about your why. Don't empty the contents just yet. Simply look at your purse, for instance. Ask yourself, "Why do I want or need this in the first place?" Consider the three causes of re-cluttering we discussed in the beginning.

The myth of more: Do you believe that more is better? Do you feel you can never have too many purses? How many purses do you currently have?

Looking outside: Do you collect purses and feel a rush when you purchase one?

Distraction attraction: Was this particular purse an impulse buy? Why exactly did you buy it?

Step Two: Direction

Step Two is about direction and perspective: where you want to go in life, how you want to be, and how you want to feel. Most of what we do and buy is driven by the belief that we will feel better as a result of doing it or buying it.

Consider these questions.

How do you want to feel by having a purse? For example, you might associate a purse with being organized, prosperous, stylish, or wealthy.

Does this particular purse contribute to that feeling?

Step Three: You Choose, You Use

Here we invoke the 80/20 rule. How often you do use this particular purse? Does it fall into the 20 percent that you use most of the time? If so, perhaps it's time to change it up.

Take a look at the rest of your purses. Select a different one that you are willing to use right now.

Step Four: Press Pause

Set an intention for yourself. Consider how much time it would take you to actually use all the purses you currently own. Let's say six months.

Make an agreement with yourself not to purchase another one during that time. Write it down. Mark it in your calendar. Plan to use your existing stuff instead.

Step Five: Lay It Out

Empty the contents of your purse, wallet, or pockets and spread them around so you can really see what you've got. Apply the 80/20 rule once again.

How much of what you are carrying around on a daily basis do you actually use? Which items would be better stored elsewhere? Which receipts are trash and which should you save for your records?

Step Six: The Six Questions

Once you've eliminated the trash and relocated items that belong elsewhere, consider the six questions for each item that remains:

 # 1. Negativity: "Are there any negative feelings or memories associated with this item? For example, are you still holding on to that keychain from an old boyfriend? If the answer is "Yes," that item is likely creating both physical and mental clutter. Get rid of it immediately by donating or recycling it. Life is too short to feel badly.

 # 2. Regularity: "Do I regularly use this item?" If the answer is "No," consider relocating, donating, or recycling it.

 # 3. Utility: "Have I used it in the last six months?" Same as above. If the answer is "No," consider relocating, donating, or recycling it.

 # 4. Contribution: "Does this item positively contribute to my life?" If the answer is "Yes," ask yourself how it adds to your life.

 # 5. Might: "Am I keeping this because I think I *might* use it at some point?" If the answer is "Yes," immediate action is required. Now's your chance to use the item. Put it in plain sight – in the most prominent part of your purse or wallet. If you haven't used it in a week, it doesn't belong in your wallet or purse.

 # 6. Guilt: "Am I keeping it out of guilt?" Maybe you spent a lot of money on that purse, so you keep it even though you don't like it or it's not very functional. Perhaps your mother-in-law gave it to you – and you never know when she might drop by. Guilt is an unhealthy reason to hold onto anything. Go immediately to Step Seven.

Step Seven: Repurpose or Recycle

For any guilt or negative association items you identified above, consider who else might enjoy them. Do the same with the items you haven't used in more than six months. Consider recycling or donating them.

Come Out of the Closet

Now that you've experienced an immediate win with your purse, wallet, or pockets, let's tackle the bedroom closet. I suggest starting with your shoes.

Step One: Awareness

This is where you examine your why. Why did you buy each pair of shoes? Why do you still have them? Keep in mind the three causes of re-cluttering we discussed earlier.

The myth of more: More is not better. More is simply more.

Looking outside: We look outside at stuff rather than at the internal feeling that's behind it. What feeling or state of being did you believe that purchase would provide?

Distraction attraction: Is your growing shoe collection covering up some unmet need? Was any of it an impulse buy?

Step Two: Direction

The idea here is to move in the direction of what feels good.

• Do you buy shoes mainly for utility or as a fashion statement?

• What feelings do you associate with your shoes?

• Does this particular pair contribute to that feeling?

This step can also refer to how your shoes physically feel when you wear them. Try them all on now. If any of them hurt your feet, consider either taking them in for repairs or donating them immediately. I personally would rather have two pairs of shoes that feel fabulous than 10 that don't fit well or are worn out.

Step Three: You Choose, You Use

After you have separated the shoes that fit from those that don't, it's time to start wearing them. This is where things get interesting. Starting today, you will wear a pair of shoes that you did not wear yesterday. At the end of the day, temporarily relocate those shoes to the other side of the closet or separate them in some way from the others. Tomorrow you will pick another pair from the unworn pile. Each day pick a new pair of shoes to wear. Continue doing this until you have cycled through them all. If you get to a pair of shoes you are not willing to wear, it is a ripe candidate for the donation pile.

Step Four: Press Pause

Impose a moratorium on new shoe purchases. If you typically buy new shoes every month or two, see if you can press the pause button for six months or more. Really stretch yourself. You likely have enough shoes to last several years. Make a game out of it. Enlist a friend who has similar shoe buying habits and challenge each other to not purchase another pair of shoes for 6-12 months.

Step Five: Lay It Out

It's easier to wear all of your shoes when you can easily see them. Do you have shoes stored in more than one closet? Are some in boxes and others in drawers? It's time to lay them all out in one place so you can see them.

Step Six: The Six Questions

Go through your shoes one by one and ask the six questions:

 # 1. Negativity: "Are there any negative feelings or memories associated with this pair of shoes?"

 # 2. Regularity: "Do I regularly wear these?"

 # 3. Utility: "Have I worn them in the last six months?"

 # 4. Contribution: "Do they positively contribute to my life?" "Do I feel good wearing them?"

 # 5. Might: "Am I keeping these because I think I *might* wear them at some point?"

 # 6. Guilt: "Am I keeping this pair out of guilt?"

When it comes to shoes and clothing, it's easy to get stuck on Question # 5 – Might. Put all the pairs you think you might wear at some point in plain sight – ideally in the most prominent part of your closet. Don't return the shoes to their boxes or drawers until you have worn them. If you haven't worn them in a month or two, consider donating them. No excuses for those special occasion shoes either. You don't have to wait for a holiday or anniversary to wear your special occasion shoes. Any random Wednesday will do. There is always something to celebrate! Get creative! Wear them around the house and feel great right now if you want to.

Step Seven: Repurpose or Recycle

Donate any shoes you that don't fit properly or that you are not willing to wear on a regular basis.

* * *

Now apply the 7-step *Free and Clear* process with the rest of your wardrobe, including your socks, underwear, and other accessories. Make a game out of wearing all your stuff!

For your clothes, I recommend creating an empty space at the furthermost end of your closet. Perhaps use an empty hanger or two to separate this area from the rest of your clothes. Tonight, put whatever you're wearing right now at the furthermost end of your closet. Tomorrow, pick new items to wear without repeating any items from yesterday. That means a different shirt and different pants, skirt, or jeans. Each day you will pick all of your clothing from the section you have not yet worn.

Keep doing this until you have cycled through all your pants, skirts, dresses, and shirts. Only repeat the "bottoms," for example, after you have worn them all once. If you get to an item you are not willing to wear, set it aside and ask yourself the six questions.

After you have worn about half of your wardrobe, you will likely have to get creative with your outfits. Start combining things you normally wouldn't. This exercise forces you to look at your clothes in a refreshing new light. Who knows…you may discover a whole new, more expressive style for yourself!

Lighten Your Living Space

Now let's move to your main living space. This could be your living room, family room, or den. This is where emotions often get the best of us. We collect knick knacks on vacation. We receive holiday, birthday, anniversary, and other special occasion gifts. Our kids give us their arts and crafts from school projects.

It's easy to see how this stuff can quickly add up.

Step One: Awareness

Take a good look around the room. Which areas offer the most potential for decluttering? Make a mental note. Now consider how your past thoughts and beliefs contributed to the contents of this room. Is there any evidence of the "more is better" belief? Are there signs of "distraction attraction" here? Simply notice what comes up.

Step Two: Direction

In this step we move in the direction of what feels good.

Sit quietly for a moment, close your eyes, and imagine your ideal living space. Forget about the contents of the room and focus on the feeling. What is the feeling that your ideal living room or family room would give you? Get into that feeling space now. Would it feel spacious? Bright? Clear? Airy? Comfy? Nurturing? Or something else? Feel this in your body. Feel that right now.

Step Three: You Choose, You Use

Once you have that feeling, it's time to take action. Open your eyes and look around the room once more. Notice how your current space makes you feel. Do a mental scan and identify the 80/20. You might want to grab a notebook for this part.

Take a look around and jot down those items you rarely use or no longer enjoy. For example, is there a chair in the corner of the room that no one ever sits in? Which books on the shelves haven't been read? Are there candles in the room that haven't been lit? What about that basket of magazines next to the couch? Or the new deck of cards still wrapped in plastic? Jot it all down.

Sidebar: A common objection I usually get right about now is this. "Not everything we buy is about utility. Some of it is worth having for the sheer beauty of it." I totally agree. So let's consider those things that are just nice to look at. How often do you actually look at your paintings on the walls or the other items that you say spark joy for you? Be honest. Again, it isn't the thing in and of itself that sparks joy. It's you who attaches the idea of joy to it. So yes, that chair in the corner might be beautiful. But did you purchase it to occasionally look at it and enjoy its beauty or to actually sit on it?

Step Four: Press Pause

Now set a goal or intention for yourself. Given the amount of rarely used items on your list, declare that you will refrain from buying any living room items for six months while you experiment with using, enjoying, and appreciating your current stuff.

Step Five: Lay It Out

Next, you'll examine your stuff to see if there are any immediate candidates for decluttering. Start with one shelf or drawer and spread its contents around.

Step Six: The Six Questions

Go over each item on that shelf or drawer and ask the six questions:

 # 1. Negativity: "Are there any negative feelings or memories associated with this item?"

 # 2. Regularity: "Do I regularly use or enjoy it?"

 # 3. Utility: "Have I used or actively enjoyed it in the last six months?"

 # 4. Contribution: "Does it positively contribute to my life?" "How?"

 # 5. Might: "Am I keeping it because I think I *might* use it at some point?"

 # 6. Guilt: "Am I keeping it out of guilt?"

Warning: When it comes to knick knacks and other living room items, it is easy to fall into a trap with Question # 1. The trap is to associate all of your stuff with a positive memory or emotion, as a way to justify keeping it. Relax! I am not suggesting you round up all your travel souvenirs or framed photos of the family and cart them off to the donation center. What I am suggesting is to consider how you might be emotionally attached to your physical stuff. If you find it very difficult to even think of parting with anything from your living room, for example, this may be why.

Remember, the stuff in and of itself has no meaning. You are the meaning maker. You attach the meaning to the stuff.

The truth is, you can generate the desired feeling with or without the stuff. Consider revisiting the "three months to live" exercise we discussed earlier. If you knew you had only three months left on the planet, how important would that item be then? How might a more spacious, uncluttered environment contribute to what you really want and how you really want to feel?

Step Seven: Repurpose or Recycle

For any negative association and guilt items, sell or donate them immediately. For knick knacks, souvenirs, kid projects, and other items that you don't actively use or enjoy but still have some feeling attached to them, consider taking a photo of them instead. That way you can store the item and the associated memory on your phone or computer – and simultaneously free up some space in your living room. For all the rest, continue the experiment of using and enjoying your stuff while pressing pause on all new purchases.

Core Kitchen

Time now to clean up the kitchen. Let's start with your food.

First, the facts. It's estimated that 30-40% of the entire food supply is wasted in the United States. That translates to more than 20 pounds of food per person per month![2] Discount and big box stores encourage and incentivize us to buy in bulk, thereby reinforcing the myth that more is better.

Don't get me wrong. There's nothing wrong with stocking up on toilet paper. You wouldn't want to run out of that. But what about that five-pound jar of pickles you bought months ago because it was a deal you couldn't pass up? Buying in large quantities can be cheaper, but only if you actually eat it all before it spoils.

You might be shocked to discover how much of your food, canned goods, spices, and sauces is already old, expired, or spoiled. Let's apply the 7-step *Free and Clear* system to your kitchen and find out.

Step One: Awareness

Examine your food habits. Why do you eat what you eat? How often do shop for food? What criteria do you use to determine what goes into your shopping cart or in your stomach? How important is nutritional content, shelf life, ease of preparation, or convenience? What are your beliefs around food? Aside from the obvious purpose of food as fuel for your body, what other meaning have you applied to certain foods?

Let's look inside your refrigerator or pantry right now. Is there any evidence of the "more is better" belief? Are there any comfort food items or foods that have very little nutritional value? Are there foods you consume primarily for entertainment, as part of a celebration, or for any reason *other than providing nutrition for your cells?*

The purpose of these questions is to bring more awareness to why you eat the way you eat – and why you buy certain foods. Start to notice your why.

Step Two: Direction

Step two is about determining what you are moving toward in life, how you want to be, and how you want to feel. For example, if your intention is to have radiant health, a fit body, and lots of energy to enjoy life to its fullest, your food choices would need to support that.

Take another look in your refrigerator and pantry. What are your current food choices supporting?

Step Three: You Choose, You Use

Be a maximizer! Eat all your food (not all at once, of course). Start by checking the expiration dates on everything you have in your pantry, refrigerator, and freezer. If anything is already a week or two past the expiration date, compost those items where possible and dispose of the rest.

Step Four: Press Pause

See how long you can go without buying any more food. Take the eat-all-your-food challenge! If you normally go to the supermarket once a week, experiment with waiting 2-3 weeks instead.

Get creative! Just because the almond butter is almost gone doesn't mean you need to run out and get another one. How about using coconut oil or olive oil instead?

And what about all those spices? Start looking for ways to add that turmeric you bought months ago to your food. Mix it up! You will likely discover some new, interesting food combinations.

Step Five: Lay It Out

This step isn't as critical when it comes to food, so there's no need to spread your food items around the kitchen. Just by virtue of pressing pause on new purchases, you will soon know exactly what you have left to eat.

Step Six: The Six Questions

Here's how the six questions apply to food.

> **# 1. Negativity:** "Are there any negative feelings associated with this item? In other words, did you buy those cheese puffs because you were having a bad day?

 # 2. Regularity: "Do I regularly use or enjoy it?" Do you keep buying the same pasta sauce, use only half of it, and then have to throw it out weeks later because mold has started to grow?

 # 3. Utility: "Have I used or actively enjoyed it in the last six months?" I personally can't imagine any foodstuff worth consuming six months after purchasing it. Even if you are stocking up and preparing for the apocalypse, it's still best to eat your stash and replace it periodically.

 # 4. Contribution: "Does it positively contribute to my life?" Common trap alert! It's easy to misinterpret this one. Revisit your intention in Step Two. If your intention is to have radiant health and vitality, those sugary or fattening comfort foods would not qualify as a positive contribution.

 # 5. Might: "Am I keeping it because I think I *might* use it?" Maybe you bought that oil, sauce, or spice because you wanted to make a certain dish – then never did. Now's your chance!

 # 6. Guilt: "Am I keeping it out of guilt?" Did you take food home from a restaurant so as not to waste it, even though you didn't want it? Did you agree to take food home from a friend or relative's house just to make the host feel good?

Step Seven: Repurpose or Recycle

Compost any food items that are spoiled or expired. For foods that do not support your desired state of health, consider donating the unopened packages or taking them to the office.

Clear Your Mental Clutter

When you simplify your physical stuff, you automatically bring more spaciousness and calm to your mind. Whether you realized it or not, each time you went through Step One (Awareness) and Step Two (Direction) in each area of your home we've discussed so far, you've cleared away some of your mental clutter.

You can use the *Free and Clear* process to declutter your head even further. Here's how:

Step One: Awareness

It's estimated that up to 70 percent of our daily thoughts are negative. It's likely that the bulk of your thoughts are the same thoughts you had yesterday. In this step, start monitoring your thoughts to see if this is true for you. Pay attention to how often you get carried away by negative or disempowering thoughts – or any thought that contains a *should*.

When you catch yourself, simply cancel that thought in your mind and replace it with a thought that feels better.

Step Two: Direction

Visualize your preferred mental state, right now. Visualize what you really want and how you want to feel. Do this several times a day. You can feel better right now by switching to a better-feeling thought or by visualizing something that feels good.

You are powerful. Dare to be aware of your power to choose.

Steps Three, Four and Five

Consider what might be contributing to your negative and repetitive thoughts. In my work with clients from all walks of life, I've noticed two common sources of mental clutter: 1) media exposure, and 2) other people. Let's consider each of these:

> **Media:** The more magazines you read and the more television you watch, the more likely you are to buy stuff you don't really need. In fact, you may not actually want it either. What you want is the feeling the new thing gives you. That feeling doesn't come from the thing. It comes from you.

> **Other People:** Despite what we would like to believe, stress isn't caused by other people. It's caused by our reaction to them. The good news is that you have complete control over your reactions.

Now, let's discover the 80/20 of the media you consume and the people you surround yourself with.

Grab a notebook and pen. Write down all forms of media you are exposed to. That means any newspapers, magazines, television shows, blogs, podcasts, and radio programs. Once you've got them all down, go through the list and identify the 20 percent you most commonly invite into your experience.

Do the same for the people in your life. Write down the names of your family members, friends, co-workers, and neighbors. Now go through the list and identify the 20 percent you spend the most time with.

Step Six: The Six Questions

Start with your list of media influences.

 # 1. Negativity: "Is the content of this newspaper or radio program primarily positive or negative?

 # 2. Regularity: "How often do I consume this form of media?

 # 3. Utility: "Have I used it in the last six months?" For example, do you have stacks of magazines you haven't read? Or do you subscribe to email newsletters that you rarely read?

 # 4. Contribution: "Does it positively contribute to my life?" This is the big one. Honestly ask yourself whether that television program, blog, or radio program adds to your life in a meaningful way.

 # 5. Might: "Am I keeping it because I think I might use it at some point?" Think unread e-zines and magazines.

 # 6. Guilt: "Am I keeping it out of guilt?"

Now move to your list of people in your life and ask the questions again.

 # 1. Negativity: "Do you have any negative feelings or unfinished business with this person? If so, consider how you might rectify the situation or change your perspective about it. How might you change your beliefs about it?

 # 2. Regularity: "Do I regularly spend time with this person?" In other words, are they part of your 80 or your 20?

 # 3. Utility: Careful with this one. Utility is not necessarily a good thing when it comes to people. Consider whether you keep someone around just because they are useful.

 # 4. Contribution: "Does this person positively contribute to my life?" "How?"

 # 5. Might: This one is not as applicable here.

 # 6. Guilt: "Am I with this person primarily out of guilt or obligation?"

Step Seven: Repurpose or Recycle

Consider who else might enjoy those magazines that no longer positively contribute to your life. Unsubscribe from the e-zines and blogs that no longer resonate with where you want to go and how you want to be.

As for the people in your life, this can be a bit trickier. Once you have identified which people don't positively contribute to your life, consider how you might spend less time with them.

Now, I realize that there are some "Negative Nellys" that you likely can't eliminate from your experience. In this case, focus on your thoughts about those people. You have absolute control over how you think and how you respond to them. Since you can't change them, consider changing your attitude instead.

Be the example!

When you become the example of mental clarity, optimism, and ease, one of two things can happen. They will either change their attitude to match your new positive state of being, or they will be repelled by the new you and will ease their way out of your experience on their own. Either way, it's a win-win!

PART THREE: NEXT STEPS

Now that you are familiar with the 7-step *Free and Clear* system, you can apply it to other areas of your home or office — such as your kitchen cabinets, your hall closet, or your email inbox. It's a flexible system. Feel free to move the steps around or modify the six questions to fit the area you are working on.

You can even simplify your cleaners and personal products using a version of this system. Download the free bonus chapters: **Clean Up Your Cleaners** and **Purge Your Personal Products** at http://KarinKiser.com/free-and-clear

Regardless of where you apply the system, pay close attention to Step One (Awareness) and Step Two (Direction). Those steps are critical for breaking the re-clutter cycle. Anyone can go through their closet and donate a bunch of clothes to charity. But to really be free and clear, it helps to ask yourself the deeper questions of why you do what you do — and where you want to go instead. There's nothing wrong with stuff. The question is, why do you *really* want it? Practice the shortcut to the desired feeling instead.

Do you want to be an accumulator or a maximizer? Do you actually want that new physical thing or the feeling you think it will provide? What's your 80/20 in other areas of your life? Does that thought, belief, or new purchase positively contribute to your life?

Just by virtue of reading this book — and asking yourself those deeper questions — you have become more mentally free and clear.

When you bring more awareness to your why — why you do what you do and think what you think — you generate more mental clarity and peace of mind. You embody your power to choose.

When you break the habit of re-cluttering, you break free of the anxiety and exasperation that excess physical clutter can provoke. You create much-needed space in your home and your head, so you can have more of what you really want in life. You are grateful for the external abundance that already surrounds you — and the internal abundance that you are at your core. You are at ease with your external physical stuff and your internal state of being. You feel open and spacious.

You are free and clear.

Wait!

Before you go, don't forget to get your FREE gifts...

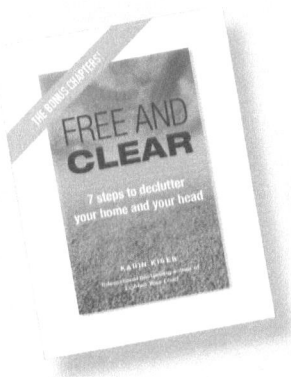

1. Clean Up Your Cleaners
2. Purge Your Personal Products

Each of these two bonus chapters will help you
on your journey to be Free and Clear.

———∞———

To get them visit:
http://KarinKiser.com/free-and-clear/

Notes

1. https://www.epa.gov/smm/advancing-sustainable-materials-management-facts-and-figures

2. https://www.usda.gov/oce/foodwaste/faqs.htm

Acknowledgements

Heartfelt appreciation goes to my readers, many of whom reported being spurred into action by the section on decluttering in my first book, *Lighten Your Load.* It was they who inspired the creation of this book.

About the Author

KARIN KISER is the founder of Radical Simplicity™, creator of the Ultimate Life and Body Reboot program, and author of the # 1 international bestseller *Lighten Your Load*. She helps people simplify and detox their lives so they can live at a higher level with more time, energy, simplicity, and ease. As a visionary and mentor, she inspires individuals around the world to greater health and happiness by teaching them to reduce the physical, mental, and emotional toxins blocking their path. She has worked with hundreds of people individually to reduce stress, lighten their load, laugh more, breathe more, and BE more.

A former corporate executive and Pilates studio owner, Karin is on a mission to help people live lives of joy, radiant health, and sustainability, for themselves and for the planet. *Free and Clear* is the second book in the Dare to Be Aware™ series. Find out more about her work at www.KarinKiser.com.

www.ingramcontent.com/pod-product-compliance
Lightning Source LLC
Chambersburg PA
CBHW050428290526
45786CB00003B/1445